The Carnivore Diet

Eating 100% Animal-Based to Lose Weight and Improve Health

By Kent Dixon

All Rights Reserved
© 2018 Kent Dixon

Table of Contents

Foreword

Evolution of the Human Diet 1

What is the Carnivore Diet and What Can You Eat? 7

Why is the Carnivore Diet Becoming Popular? 14

Potential Benefits of the Carnivore Diet 16

Potential Risks of the Carnivore Diet 21

The Importance of Nutrients 26

Author's Note 30

A Note on Gut Health 31

History of Animal-Based Diets 34

Ten Day Get Started Meal Plan 41

How to Keep Costs Down 48

Wrapping It Up 51

Making the Meals 54

Additional Resources 69

Foreword

What should I eat?

A common and seemingly simple question that many people ask themselves every day. Yet, the answer is as elusive as ever.

Over the years the link between diet and health has been explored with growing popularity and interest, to the point where individuals and organizations have now created entire industries around the idea. This process has inevitably led to many varying opinions on what a proper diet should look like. What nutrients are needed? How much protein is necessary? Is all fat bad? Should we be taking vitamins? Which ones?

The answers to those questions seem to change with the seasons, leaving the average consumer striding defeated and confused into the pastry section of their local supermarket. With advertisements and health experts pointing consumers in all imaginable directions, it can be tough to know where to turn.

Some health experts now advocate for a 100% plant-based diet, more commonly known as vegetarian.

Others simply suggest a balanced diet of meat, plants and grains is essential to proper health.

Recently, a growing number of people have been exploring the idea of eating a 100% animal-based diet, or as it has been more cleverly named: The Carnivore Diet.

Crazy...right?

Only meat? No vegetables? No Fruit? That goes against almost everything we've been told.

Well, turns out it might not actually be all that crazy. People everywhere are continuing to report drastic benefits from switching to this way of eating, ranging from simple weight loss and increased energy levels to decreasing inflammation and resolved autoimmune disorders in the body. This might seem a bit counterintuitive to most, at least it was for me at first. How does eating only meat make you healthier?

This book will look to break down all the benefits and risks associated with eating a 100% animal-based diet. It will also offer research based insight into nutrition and diet in general, and most importantly, try to provide you with some clear information so that you can have an answer the next time you possibly find yourself asking...what should I eat?

Disclaimer

I'm not a doctor, dietician, or nutritionist.

To the contrary, I obtained my Bachelor's Degree in Marketing with a specialization in consumer behaviour and market research; a pursuit that cultivated in me a healthy sense of curiosity and an inclination to research concepts rather thoroughly. I also just happen to be fascinated by health and nutrition, and have been experimenting with diet quite extensively over the past decade, so this book seemed like a natural fit.

This book is not meant to be medical advice, or to tell you what you should eat or do. The information in this book is meant to provide you with a starting point to further explore what types of diets and eating patterns work best for you as an individual. You should always consult a professional health practitioner before embarking on any serious personal changes.

P.S. Any studies or articles referenced within this book will be linked for your convenience in the Additional Resources chapter.

Evolution of the Human Diet

To answer the question of what we should be eating today it might help to look back on what we used to eat in the past. Understanding the diets that we—as humans—have typically consumed over the course of history allows us to gain insight into which elements of our diet may or may not be necessary for optimal health.

How has our diet changed over the millennia? Why did those changes occur and what impact did it have on our evolution? I won't go into every detail imaginable, but I will try to touch upon enough to give you a solid foundation (stick with me here).

Now, with that in mind, let's wind the evolutionary clock back. All the way back.

The anatomically modern human (Homo sapiens) evolved from our Hominin ancestors over the course of roughly 3 million years. Now, considering that 3 million years ago humans weren't exactly writing cookbooks and keeping meal journals, if we want to know what they were eating we have to look at their diet through a different mechanism: Comparative morphology. Essentially, we can look at how the human form changed and "morphed" over the millennia and compare that alongside other related organisms with similar anatomical features whose diets are well established. If that sounds complicated, I promise it isn't.

For example, our earliest ancestor, Australopithecus, had a much larger lower jawbone than we have today. Why? Well, we can look to gorillas for an explanation. Gorillas, just like Australopithecus, have a large lower jawbone. They require that larger jawbone to crush and chew the vast amount of dense plant matter that makes up their vegetarian diet.

This is where Comparative morphology comes in. That leads us to assume that Australopithecus would have used its larger lower jaw bone to crush a primarily plant based diet, similar to that of the Gorilla. See? Pretty straightforward. Let's move on.

As human evolution stretched on our lower jaw bones gradually decreased in size while our brains increased in size. While that was happening we also experienced a shortening in the length of our gut. What does that all translate to in terms of diet? We can look to the omnivorous chimpanzee for some answers.

Chimpanzees, when compared with our previously mentioned gorilla, have a more slender lower jaw bone, larger brain and shorter gut length. This is largely chalked up to the fact that chimpanzees, unlike gorillas, enjoy a diet of insects and small animals in addition to plants.

What does a transition from a strictly plant to meat-based diet have to do with jaw bones, brain size and gut length? Well, the argument being made by scientists is that meat was more easily chewable, resulting in less of a need for a powerful lower jaw bone to grind up tough plants. By eating the more calorie-dense meat as opposed to the low-quality plant diet, more energy is taken in to help fuel a larger brain. A reduction in the amount of bulky plant fiber and the addition of more easily digestible diet resulted in the shortening of the gut length. This also had the bonus effect of freeing up some of the precious energy being used by the previously larger gut, which could then be soaked up by the energy-greedy brain. By way of this theory, many argue it was the addition of meat to our diets that propelled us along our heightened evolutionary path.

Now, fast-forward a few million years and we land at another major shift in the human diet with the advent of large-scale agriculture roughly 10,000 years ago.

Agriculture allowed humans to cultivate land and develop sustainable crops to provide a reliable food source from a single plot of land. This seemed an improvement from the previously unpredictable lifestyle of hunter gatherer tribes, where no meal was ever guaranteed.

Over the course of the past 10,000 years agriculture has grown to take a more and more prominent role in our society, eventually landing at present day wherein the main component of most individual's diet is now comprised of the yields from agriculture. This has slowly resulted in a typical diet being increasingly comprised of carbohydrates as opposed to fats and proteins.

Keep in mind that while 10,000 years may seem like a very long time for this shift to occur—and you might think humans would be able to slowly get used to the change in diet and evolve over that time—on the evolutionary clock, it's barely one second.

Adaptations and changes that occur in our body can take hundreds of thousands if not millions of years to occur. Evolution is slow. To put things in perspective, we have existed in our current form—Homo sapiens—for roughly 250,000-300,000 years. That means our entire body, including the digestive system, is roughly the same as it was almost 300,000 years ago. This has led many to wonder if our body is setup to run better on a diet and lifestyle that more closely resembles that of our hunter-gatherer ancestors. A diet from before the advent of large-scale agriculture, arguing that these dietary changes that have occurred over the past 10,000 years have been too recent on the evolutionary time scale for the human genome to have fully adapted; Our slow rate of change and adaptation may not enable us to adjust alongside such a drastically quick change in the types of nutrients we put in our body, potentially resulting in a wide array of health issues.

More recently on this 10,000 year journey of agriculture and human diet, another shift occurred. This shift was the result of an innovation in the way we processed our grains. Riveting, I know. You see, historically to make flour you would take a wheat grain and simply grind and crush it between two spinning slabs of rock to make what we would call "whole grain" flour—cleverly named because we use the whole grain, every part of it. However, the bread that the whole grain flour made was typically pretty dense and hard to chew, and people quickly found out that if you separated parts of the wheat grain you could get a softer flour, and in turn softer bread. I'm talking of course about "white flour". The process to get white flour is actually quite simple: remove the bran and germ from the grain and you're left with the part that is mostly starch. While it may be simple, that process proved to be rather labour intensive and as such was expensive, so white flour wasn't widely available to the average person in the past. This is where that innovation I mentioned earlier comes in. The roller mill. The roller mill was introduced into agriculture in late 19th century and essentially functioned to shake and roll the wheat so that the bran and germ would fall away, and you would only be left with starchy part. Now automatable and no longer a labour intensive process, white flour became much more affordable and accessible to the general public. Soon, everyone was eating it.

Almost overnight, this invention completely changed the way the average person consumed their grains and carbohydrates. Turns out that most of the nutritional value of the grain (the vitamins and minerals in this case) lies within the bran and germ that the roller milling sheds off. So, not only have we recently—in evolutionary terms—added in a very large amount of grains into our diet with the advent of agriculture, we've now taken away much of the nutritional value within those grains by creating white flour.

Now, if that idea I mentioned earlier of slow anatomical adjustments holds up, and we really haven't fully adapted to the change in our diet that happened 10,000 years ago, what level of impact could these additional changes within the last few hundred years be having on our bodies?

Studies have shown that over the past 300 years the average American diet has had a staggering increase in sugar consumption. In the 1700s the average American consumed roughly 4 pounds of sugar in a year. By the 1800s that had increased to approximately 22 pounds. By 2009, 50 percent of Americans were consuming close to 180 pounds of sugar in a year.

In the spirit of transparency, I'll point out that there have been many studies on this that all derive different levels of consumption for each time period. Some say we only consumed 2 pounds—not 4—of sugar in the 1700s. Others also say that we consume 150 pounds a year now, while others assume much higher.

Regardless of what the numbers really are, the result is the same. Whether it went from 2 pounds a year to 150, or 6 pounds a year to 110, it was an exponential explosion of sugar into our digestive system over a very short window of roughly 300 years. Studies have now been done to look at the potential link between our increase in sugar consumption and the increased rates of many common diseases. One in particular was done over the course of 15 years, and had one group of participants acquire 17-21% of their calories from sugar, while the other group only had 8% of their calories from sugar. The results concluded that the group with the higher consumption levels of sugar had a 38% higher risk of dying from cardiovascular disease when compared to the lower group. Other studies have shown links between high levels of added sugar and increased risks for type 2 diabetes, hypertension (AKA high blood-pressure), weight gain and obesity.

The reason so many Americans—and I'll note the figures are similar in the UK—are consuming more sugar now than ever before, is largely due to the fact that sugar seems to be in almost everything nowadays.

Do yourself a favour and take a few minutes next time you're at the grocery store and venture into the middle isles. Pick up a few things off the shelves here and there and read some of the nutritional labels and ingredients. There are a lot of products out there that you naturally assume wouldn't have a need for added sugar—pasta sauce comes to mind—that list sugar as an ingredient. Almost all processed foods are packed with added sugars to ensure they taste as good as possible and to keep you coming back for more. Foods that in the past would have had little to no sugar are now packed with all different types of sugars and sweeteners.

This trend to add sugar into everything—amongst a few other factors—is a large contributor to the rise of sugar levels in the average American diet. This has made it more important than ever to "watch what you eat", making sure to read the nutritional labels on the backs of foods to ensure you aren't consuming needless amounts of added sugars. Now, this is easier said than done for most individuals who follow a traditional "western" diet, as the bulk of their diet is typically made up of a high amount of processed foods. However, for individuals following a 100% animal based diet, it's quite a simple task to achieve.

Many view the carnivore diet as a way to wind back the clock and eat a diet that aligns itself more naturally with our body's needs. Cutting out the breads, sugars and processed foods that have become so prolific in the past few centuries in favour of a food that our body has known for millions of years.

Is this the best option for everyone? Can we truly thrive on a diet solely of meat like these people are pronouncing? I think those are interesting questions that deserve some answers, or at the very least to be explored a bit more thoroughly.

So, without further introduction, let's take a look at the carnivore diet.

What is the Carnivore Diet and What Can You Eat?

Although the diet title doesn't leave much to the imagination, I'll break it down as simply as possible:

Eat only animal products.
Don't eat plants.

The above two sentences mean that you won't eat any vegetables, fruits, nuts, seeds, legumes or starches. Some proponents of the diet allow for the consumption of dairy, however, others do not as lactose is a sugar. More on this later.

This diet is also commonly referred to as the "zero-carb" diet, due to the fact that it essentially limits your carbohydrate intake to zero. There are a few exceptions to this, as there are small amounts of carbohydrates in some animal products that are incorporated in the diet, but those are generally acceptable.

Which brings up the questions: what all can you eat on the carnivore diet?

Here's a list to get you going:

- Beef
- Chicken
- Eggs
- Lamb
- Buffalo
- Elk
- Pork

- Fish
- Turkey
- Duck
- Goat
- Snake
- Alligator
- Frog
- Seafood (Crab, lobster, oysters, shrimp, etc.)
- Insects
- Organ Meat (Liver is the most common)
- Dairy (Optional)

That might not be a comprehensive list of every type of meat on the planet, but for the sake of the carnivore diet those are all you'll need. To be honest, you'll really only need a few.

Off the start, most people transitioning to a 100% animal-based diet try to eat as diverse a selection as possible. Maybe some chicken one day, beef the next, throw in some lamb and turkey; variety is important, right?

While I agree that variety can be important in most diets, the majority of individuals are going to find themselves shifting to the same staple meat that most on the carnivore diet prioritize. Beef.

As you cut out other food groups from your diet, you are also cutting out the calories that those foods contributed to your diet. The fattier cuts of beef are the most effective at staving off hunger, and will keep you feeling full the longest. That is why most on the carnivore diet find themselves primarily eating ribeye steaks, as it is one of the most nutritionally and calorically dense meat options with a high fat content. Steering towards fattier cuts of meat will ensure you get enough calories in the day and can maintain proper energy levels.

What about liquids? What should you be drinking when it comes to the carnivore diet? This list is a much shorter than the previous index of meats:

- Water
- Bone broth
- Black Coffee (Optional)
- Tea (Optional)

That's it.

No alcohol, soda, or juice.

My list is actually a bit longer than some carnivore dieters would accept, as some people like to use a simple little equation to sum up the diet:

Meat + Water = Carnivore Diet.

That equation doesn't leave any room for other liquids, but I have decided to include a few anyways.

I added bone broth to the list because while you might not think too highly of trading in your glass of orange juice for some bone broth first thing in the morning, it's a great way to add in some important nutrients to your diet. Nutrients which, as I'll explain in a bit, can be very important.

Now, before I continue on explaining why you should care about bone broth, it's important to define what bone broth is, because it might be different than what you think. At least I know it was for me. I thought I could just go to the store and buy some beef or chicken broth off the shelf and be good to go. What I found was there seems to be three distinct types of "broth" that people can buy: Plain broth, stock and bone broth.

Plain Broth: This is simply the carton of broth you would most likely head out and buy at your typical supermarket. It's a mix of vegetables, seasoning, chicken or beef bones, all simmered for a relatively short amount of time.

Stock: Essentially the same as plain broth, only difference being that the recipe is usually a bit heavier in the bone category and the ingredients simmer for longer. This translates into more nutrients being extracted from the bones.

Bone Broth: This is the good stuff. Main difference between bone broth and the previous two types, simmer time. Bone broth will have even more bones than the other types, and will simmer for up to 48 hours in some cases. The longer simmer time extracts all the gelatin and minerals from the bones to give you the biggest nutritional bang-for-your-buck.

Despite those differences, if you were to read the nutritional information on the back of a each pack of broth, first off it might not seem like they're all that different. Second, you might not be all that impressed. Relatively low in calories, no vitamin A or C, and negligible amounts of calcium and iron.

If it doesn't have any of those nutrients, what does it have? Glad you asked.

While nutritional labels are usually a great place to start for information on a product, they don't always tell the whole tale. In this case, they don't mention the amino acids or minerals that make bone broth so nutritionally valuable.

No matter the type of bone used to make it, bone broth contains high levels of both collagen and gelatin. Both of these proteins break down into a wide array of amino acids that have shown to aid human health in a number of different ways. Rather than list every single amino acid in bone broth, I'll stick to a few you might care about:

Arginine

Arginine or L-arginine has been shown to dilate blood vessels, which aids in nutrient transport within your body. That translates into more nutrients and protein to your muscles which aids in muscle growth, increased blood flow to your heart which has been shown to improve your cardiovascular systems performance, and improved blood flow to a few other regions on your body which can in turn have a positive impact on your sexual health.

Glycine

Although glycine has been shown to have numerous health benefits, one of the most commonly touted is its ability to aid with sleep. Glycine acts primarily on N-methyl-D-aspartate (NMDA) receptors, and is believed to reduce or inhibit muscle activity during rapid eye movement (REM) sleep, and to reduce core temperature, both of which can aid in achieving a more restful sleep.

Proline

Proline helps the body to do a number of beneficial functions: form collagen, form connective tissue, regenerate cartilage, repair joints, and repair skin damage.

Although it might not sound like a huge benefit, proline also helps to improve your gut health (more on the importance of gut health in Chapter 9) and can even treat leaky gut syndrome.

Glutamine

Glutamine is the most abundant amino acid in our body. Although our bodies naturally produce glutamine, we require so much that we typically have to obtain more through our diet.

Glutamine is stored in the muscles and has been shown to aid in muscle recovery, and prevent muscle depletion. Just like proline, it also helps to regulate gut health and prevent leaky gut syndrome.

So, those are all the reasons I decided to throw bone broth on the list. It falls under the definition of "animal-based" and if you're switching over to the carnivore diet to try and be healthier, you can't argue with the potential benefits.

Now, as promised earlier, I said I would talk a bit about dairy and the potential role it can play in a 100% animal-based diet.

While most will avoid it, dairy seems to be an acceptable non-meat food source for some individuals on the carnivore diet. The dairy is typically limited to the full fat range: cheese, ghee, yogurt, butter and heavy cream.

The reason that most avoid dairy is due to the high prevalence of allergies. Studies have shown that close to 75% of the world's population have an inability to break down lactose. You might have heard of this…lactose intolerant? It's much more common than people might think.

That being said, every individual processes dairy differently. Some might be fine with a small amount of cheese added in to their diet, others may not be.

In the end, I personally believe that the best course of action would be to cut out dairy entirely once you are fully committed to the carnivore diet. Slowly reintroduce dairy after a while to see how you feel, and evaluate from there. This way you can compare how you felt with dairy included in the diet, and without.

Why is the Carnivore Diet Becoming Popular?

As of the time this is being written, the carnivore diet seems to be gaining significant popularity in the media. This is largely due to the pronounced benefits that so many people are attributing to the diet. The internet is ripe with personal stories of people losing weight and feeling better than they ever have after switching to the carnivore diet. A few of those stories in particular are making their rounds with the masses. This has thrust the carnivore diet into the spotlight, and public awareness surrounding this 100% animal-based way of eating has increased dramatically.

Most notably, Canadian professor, writer, and public figure, Jordan Peterson came out to say he was eating an all meat diet. He started following the diet largely due to the success his daughter, Mikhaila Peterson, was having with the 100% meat only diet treating a host of autoimmune issues she was experiencing, such as: idiopathic arthritis, depression, and various skin complications.

Seeing the benefits his daughter was experiencing from the new eating protocol, Jordan decided to transition to the diet himself and see if he experienced any of the same general health benefits. He started eating only ribeye steaks and drinking water, and has since reported a wide array of improvements in not only his physical well-being, but his mental health as well.

It is important to note that while there are many stories of individuals experiencing significant benefits from an all-meat diet it is merely anecdotal evidence and shouldn't be relied upon as treatment advice. Treat it as you would a friend recommending a new, rather unstudied diet to you based off their positive experiences with it. Just because there aren't any studies done on the subject doesn't mean it is inherently bad advice, it just means you should proceed with caution.

Another public advocate for the carnivore diet is Shawn Baker, an orthopedic surgeon and high-performance athlete. Dr. Baker started on the carnivore diet in an effort to improve his physical performance, prevent age-related diseases, and reduce joint pain. After noticing significant benefits he ended up continuing with the diet. His diet, just like Jordan Peterson's, is almost exclusively made up of ribeye steaks.

If you do a bit of research on these people on your own, or even just throw their name in a Google search, you'll inevitably be met by a wealth of interviews and articles where they discuss the myriad benefits they claim to be experiencing as a result of this diet. Some of those benefits more drastic than others.

So, what are these benefits that seem to have everyone heading out to go buy themselves some steak?

Let's take a look.

Potential Benefits of the Carnivore Diet

If I gave you one guess as to what the most common reason dieters started their new eating regime is, I bet most would guess correctly: To lose weight.

Weight Loss or Weight Management

Maybe one of the most talked about benefits of the carnivore diet is its ability to help with weight loss. Individuals debate the reasons as to why the weight loss occurs, however, the most common school of thought references the ketogenic diet for a possible answer. This is because the ketogenic diet shares one important similarity with the carnivore diet: the main source of calories comes from fats as opposed to carbohydrates.

Whenever the body requires energy and carbohydrates are not available it will start to increase ketone levels and go into a state of ketosis—hence the name "ketogenic" diet. The longer the body is without carbohydrates the higher the ketone levels will become. This is because ketones are converted into energy when our preferred fuel source, carbohydrates, is not available in our system. Although there are a wide array of reported benefits to using ketones for energy and being in a state of ketosis, I'll focus on just one. Weight loss.

A study was done that looked at the efficiency of three different diets in achieving weight loss amongst a sample group of 322 moderately obese people. The study was performed over a period of two years, with the 322 participants all being randomly assigned one of three diets: low-fat, restricted-calorie; Mediterranean, restricted-calorie; low-carbohydrate, non-restricted-calorie. 95.4% of participants were still adhering to their diets at the one year mark, and at the end of two years that had dropped to 84.6%. The results showed that the low-carb, non-restricted-calorie diet had the highest percentage of participants with detectable urinary ketones as well as the highest average weight loss (4.7kg).

Another study looked at the impact a low-carbohydrate diet had on weight loss in comparison to a "conventional" weight loss diet. It took 132 obese adults and randomly assigned them to either diet. The rules for one diet were to limit carbohydrates to below 30 grams per day, the other to reduce daily calories by 500 with less than 30% of calories from fat.

The results showed that at the end of one year the patients on the low-carbohydrate diet experienced "more favourable" outcomes. Although the weight loss levels were admittedly close between the groups, the low-carbohydrate group did lose more weight on average.

Another popular theory as to why weight loss occurs on the carnivore diet is that you will simply eat less, and therefore take in less calories. Eating fatty cuts of meat is particularly satiating, which means that you can typically feel full even while eating less food. This inevitably leads to consuming less calories. One of the most important aspects of weight loss on any diet is something called "caloric deficit". Simply put, you want to burn more calories than you take in. If your body is spending more energy than you are consuming, you will lose weight. Plain and simple. Moving to the carnivore diet will drastically reduce how many calories you consume each day, inevitably making it easier to lose weight.

Decreased Inflammation

As the prevalence of inflammatory diseases continues to rise, many individuals have been investigating the role that a high carbohydrate diet may have on inflammation levels in the body.

A recent study was done that examined if altering the diet of individuals with Type 2 Diabetes, an inflammatory disease, could help modulate their levels of inflammation.

The test group was broken in half, one group was prescribed a traditional low fat diet while the other was to eat a low carb diet. They collected test results at the beginning to establish a baseline, then again at six months to measure any changes.

The results came back to show that the group on the low carb diet experienced an improvement in their inflammatory state, while the group on the low fat diet did not. The low carb group also had beneficial effects on their glycemic control, while once again, the low fat group did not.

Another study was conducted that looked at the impact a low carb, high fat diet can have on inflammation amongst obese individuals. Similar to the aforementioned study, the subjects were divided into two groups with one prescribed a high fat, low carbohydrate diet and the other a low fat, high carbohydrate diet.

The study spanned twelve weeks and the results showed that between the two groups, the low carb, high fat group had greater improvements in blood lipids and systemic inflammation.

Seeing as how eating 100% animal-based will all but eliminate your carbohydrate intake, it stands to reason that it in turn may help to reduce inflammation in the body as a result.

Increased Testosterone

Although testosterone is mainly thought of as the "male" hormone (estrogen being it's female counterpart), it regulates a wide array of bodily functions in both men and women. Testosterone plays an important role in: sex drive, muscle growth, bone mass, brain function, and even mood.

Testosterone can naturally decrease as we age, but it is not uncommon for some individuals to have lower levels of the hormone simply due to various lifestyle and diet choices. Luckily, there are many ways to increase hormone production for those that suffer from low testosterone, one of them being diet.

One study looked at the impact a high fat, low fibre diet can have on hormone levels when compared to a typical low fat, high fibre diet. The study was performed on 43 healthy men between the ages of 19 and 56. They were each to eat a high fat, low fibre diet for 10 weeks, then go back to their regular diet for two weeks to reset, and then eat a low-fat, high-fibre diet for another 10 weeks. The participant's hormone levels were tested throughout the diet in order to assess any changes.

The results showed that in both the plasma and urine tested, testosterone levels were higher in the men during the high fat, low fibre diet—by roughly 15%—when compared to levels while on the low-fat, high-fibre diet.

A diet that is 100% animal-based is going to be much higher in fats than in fibre, and so if the results of the study hold up, one can assume that eating that way will lead to an increase in testosterone levels.

Simplicity

No one likes having to constantly think about the nutrients in their food and add up how many grams of carbs and fats they are getting at every meal.

It can be exhausting constantly having to read labels to ensure a product isn't going to ruin your diet. Or having to track how many points each item in your meals are worth to make sure you don't go over your daily limit. Your diet shouldn't require you to use a spreadsheet and a meal journal to make sure you are staying on track.

Eating 100% animal-based takes all the frustrating and tiresome diet calculations out of your life.

When compared with other eating protocols, eating a 100% animal-based diet is refreshingly simple. No more counting macronutrients every meal, or adding up weight watchers points. The only thought you need to have is, is this 100% animal based?

Now, this might not seem like a very big benefit to some people, but to others it will make a world of difference. Not just in the way they approach their diet, but in the way they approach their life. Just think about how much time and energy you spend making decisions surrounding your diet.

What should I make for breakfast today? Lunch? Supper? Questions that, for some, have easy answers, while for others, can be a point of much frustration and indecision. Especially for people who lead busy, hectic lives, following a diet where decisions are kept to a minimum can be a welcomed change.

Plus, no more grocery lists that look like a two-part novel.

Potential Risks of the Carnivore Diet

All diets have risks and downsides. You could be impacted by all of them, or none of them. It really all depends on the individual.

When you have a population as diverse as we do on this planet, there are bound to be individuals that respond better or worse to the same exact diet. Every person will have some level of variance in their ability to process different types of foods and nutrients, and in turn can react differently to the same diet. Even small differences in genetics and lifestyle can impact how a person will respond to one way of eating versus another.

This variance in response is why it is important to address any potential risks that may arise with a change in diet, but is also the reason each individual must take these risks with a grain of salt. The same holds true for the aforementioned benefits. Just because one person—or even a thousand—experience a given result from a diet, doesn't mean you will too. With that in mind, here are some of the potential downsides to the carnivore diet.

Lack of Long-Term Studies

Although there are some reports of some individuals claiming to have been following the carnivore diet for over 20 years, those reports are few and far between and typically anecdotal in nature. There has been virtually no clinical research into the long-term impact the carnivore diet can have on an individual. Any evidence being reported in the popular media (including in this book) is either largely based upon personal stories, or on studies that evaluate comparable mechanisms and elements with the carnivore diet.

This lack of scientific research into the long-term impacts opens up the door for a wide variety of risks down the line. While you can find a wealth of blogs and articles online and read all about the benefits individuals are experiencing, at the end of the day they lack scientific validity and need to be taken for what they are: personal stories.

There is, however, a small amount of studies that examine the impact of eating an almost 100% animal-based diet, but in comparison to the research that has been done on other diets, the literature is rather thin.

Now, this isn't to say that just because a library of clinical studies doesn't yet exist that the diet will automatically have negative health implications in the long run. We really don't know either way. For the time being, all it means is that we lack a full set of resources to help us make a perfectly informed decision. Until those resources exist, we are left to piece together personal anecdotes and studies that look at comparable diets and nutritional mechanisms in an effort to paint the best picture we can of the effects this diet may have.

Potential Kidney Issues

Studies have shown that in individuals with kidney disease, a high-protein diet can negatively impact kidney function. In healthy individuals there is little to no impact on their kidneys. Considering the carnivore diet is obviously very high in protein, this may be a potential concern for some individuals.

The study looked at the common claim that too much protein stresses the kidneys, and examined the role dietary protein can have on kidney function, as well as kidney disease. It studied individuals that consumed a high protein diet, which they defined as 1.5 grams of protein, per kilogram of body weight, per day. This would equate to roughly twice the recommended dietary allowance of protein for the average individual.

The findings concluded that individuals with pre-existing kidney disease should tread carefully with high protein intake levels, however, in a healthy individual there were no adverse impacts to the kidney when following a high-protein diet. Plainly put, if you already have kidney issues the carnivore diet could make them worse. If you're a healthy individual with properly functioning kidneys, based off the results of this individual study, an increase in your protein intake will not negatively impact kidney health.

Nutrient Deficiencies

One of the most commonly cited risks when discussing the pros and cons of eating a 100% animal-based diet—or any diet for that matter—is the potential for nutrient deficiencies. Many people point out that there are a few vitamins and minerals that we simply can't obtain from eating a solely meat based diet. Most notably, Vitamin C.

If you eat an all meat diet you won't be able to get anywhere near the recommended dietary allowance (RDA) of Vitamin C that most health organizations will say you need. Depending on which organization you subscribe to, the range can be anywhere from 60-120 mg/day of Vitamin C to maintain optimal health. According to one study in the American Journal of Clinical Nutrition, not meeting these requirements, and going below a 46 mg/day threshold is said to lead to a deficiency disease called scurvy.

Scurvy is a disease that historically used to be quite common amongst one particular class of individuals: pirates and sailors. Seeing as how ships would typically spend long, extended periods of time at sea, crew members didn't exactly have the luxury of a eating fresh foods. All the perishable foods such as fruits and vegetables had to be eaten first thing before they went rotten, and thereafter the crew would typically be left to eat a diet largely void of Vitamin C. This lead to a disease called scurvy, and in turn a host of terrible symptoms. Loss of teeth, swollen gums, slow-healing wounds, severe and easy bruising, bleeding into joints and muscles, and much more. If left untreated long enough, the combination of all these symptoms could reach a level where the individual would eventually die from complications.

As you can imagine, scurvy is now much less prominent in the modern era. Besides a few rare cases, for the most part individuals follow a diet that provides them adequate levels of vitamin C, and keeps them far away from the dangers of this popular disease of the 1700s.

If lack of vitamin C intake can lead to a disease with such terrible symptoms, eating a diet that delivers negligible amounts of vitamin C seems like a pretty big risk to take. Yet, there are anecdotal reports of individuals following a carnivorous diet and not experiencing any nutritional deficiencies or any symptoms of scurvy and maintaining seemingly good health. There is even one study, albeit quite old, where two men volunteered to live off only meat for an entire year so that researchers could study the impact of the diet on their health. This might be one of the only long-term(ish) studies that has been done on the effects of eating a meat only diet, and the results showed that after the full year neither men were experiencing any nutrient deficiencies—or any negative health impacts for that matter.

Some individuals have theorized that this may be a result of the body needing less vitamin C when on a lower carbohydrate diet, and that the body becomes more efficient at processing vitamin C when carbohydrate intake is lowered. Keep in mind this is not a widely studied theory, but it could explain why people aren't getting sick when eating only meat. I'll explain the logic behind this a bit in the next chapter.

Another idea put forth is that the recommended daily allowances are simply wrong. The thought process being that since they are based off what an individual on a standard diet would need, they aren't accurate when if you follow a diet that is drastically different than the one used to calculate the RDAs.

While neither of these ideas have been fully accepted by the scientific community, they do bring up interesting points concerning the idea of recommended dietary allowances for nutrients. How were these levels derived? What are they based off? Most importantly, how do we know if they are correct?

The Importance of Nutrients

Our body needs 13 different vitamins to function properly each day. How much of each of those vitamins we need can depend on a couple different things: age, body composition, physical activity level, etc. The amounts each person is going to need will even change just solely based off their individual genetic makeup and their ability to process certain vitamins more or less efficiently.

Most people don't typically keep track of the exact levels of each vitamin and nutrient they are taking in each and every day, or how much is even in the foods they are consuming. This is where the ease of recommended dietary allowances (RDA) come in, or percentage of daily value (DV). I imagine almost everyone in the developed world is pretty familiar with what both of those terms are. They have most likely been on the back of pretty much every food package you've opened since you were little. You turn over the food package to read the nutritional label and you see a bunch of percentages beside the vitamins and nutrients. For example, you might check the nutritional label on a bottle of orange juice and see that it has 100% of the "Daily Value" or "DV" for Vitamin C, 0% for Iron, 25% Vitamin D, so on and so forth. A lot of people place a lot of importance on these percentages, and use them as a trusted guideline when deciding on what they consume and what is healthy.

That being said, it might be important to understand what these recommended dietary allowances and daily values actually are, because despite what most might think, the aren't talking about the same thing.

The recommended dietary allowance is developed by the Institute of Medicine to outline nutrient intake standards that will ensure normal body functioning. Essentially, it's a recommendation that factors in age and gender to give you a pretty good idea of what levels of nutrients an average person should be consuming in order to maintain good health.

The recommended dietary allowances are updated rather frequently, and are generally accepted as pretty accurate for the average individual. The daily values on the other hand are developed by the US Food and Drug Administration (FDA) and provide a much less accurate picture because they are simply based off what a person needs when following a standard 2,000 calorie, Western diet and do not adjust for age or sex. On top of that, most of the daily values haven't been updated since 1968. Now you might be thinking that following the recommended dietary allowances as opposed to the daily values might be the better option if you're looking to stay healthy. But, even the recommended dietary allowances have a few shortcomings.

One study goes into some pretty nitty gritty details on why the recommended dietary allowances aren't perfect, and some of the challenges faced when setting these guidelines. Some of those noted challenges in setting the standards are: a lack of dose-response data for some nutrients (which measures the variation in response to different levels of dosages), and the lack of long-term studies on either humans or animals that have been undertaken. And as I alluded to earlier, the recommended dietary allowances were developed based off a Western diet—a diet typically very high in carbohydrates. The authors of the study go on to point out that there is even a lack of understanding surrounding the interaction of different nutrients with one another, and the potential variability in responses. Meaning that changes in some nutrient levels could impact how other nutrients interact and are processed by the body, which in turn could impact how much of each nutrient is required for optimal health. So, while the recommended dietary allowances can be a good general guideline for health if you're following the standard Western diet, they aren't exactly perfect if you follow a different way of eating.

Now, this isn't to say that the recommended dietary allowances are completely useless for someone who follows a diet that differs from the standard Western diet. It simply means that it hasn't been studied enough to know what the proper nutrient levels are, or how they might change alongside a shift in diet. A change in diet could have no impact on the nutrients our body requires, or it could have a drastic impact, we just don't know yet.

One thing we do know, however, is that the absorption of some vitamins and minerals can limit the absorption of others. This is why some people think that removing carbohydrates from the diet could impact how efficiently our body absorbs Vitamin C, and in turn require less of it. For example, excess intake of vitamin A can inhibit our body's ability to absorb vitamin K, not taking in enough Zinc can inhibit vitamin A activity, and Vitamin D helps our body to more efficiently absorb calcium. There is a diverse and complicated relationship between all vitamins and nutrients that I am not even going to pretend to fully understand. But it is evident that as levels of some nutrients change, our body's ability to process others changes in kind. This means that as our diets and nutrient intakes change, there is a possibility that there will be a cascade effect in our bodies where some nutrients are processed more efficiently and others less efficiently. This is getting back to the idea that I brought up earlier concerning vitamin C.

How does this relate to the carnivore diet and eating a 100% animal-based diet? Well, first off since the diet is so drastically different from the standard western diet it might stand to reason that the recommended dietary allowances set forth for the standard diet might not apply. Our bodies may adjust the efficiency at which we process nutrients as we alter our dietary intake, so going well below the RDAs might not be as big an issue as some make it out to be. Proponents of the carnivore diet stand quite strongly behind the belief that humans can obtain all their required nutrients from a solely animal-based diet. Without supplementation. At the end of the day, since there hasn't been many studies done on this topic, so it's important to tread carefully when making assumptions. Like I mentioned at the start of this book, I'm not a nutritionist or a scientist, merely someone who is interested in the intricacies of diet and its impacts on the human body.

Seeing as how there is a lack of clinical studies, many have now turned to anthropological means to try and understand the nutritional and health implications of surviving on an solely animal-based diet. Societies and groups of people in the past—and a few still today—have survived on nearly 100% animal-based diets for decades and sometimes centuries. Examining these societies and people might be able to help us understand the implications of existing on such a diet for a long period of time, and possibly provide a window into the long-term health effects it could have.

Author's Note

If you've made it this far into the book I'd like to interject for a moment before we continue on. First off, I'd just like to say thank you for purchasing this book and taking the time to read it, I know you had many other options and I appreciate you choosing this one. Now, with this being one of my first published works, I would greatly appreciate your feedback on what you think so far.

Have you found any value in what I've laid out for you? Have I maybe ignited a spark of curiosity in you to further pursue some aspect of nutrition and diet? Do you think someone else might find it interesting?

At the end of the day I started this project in an effort to not only try and help people, but to also learn and grow my skills as a writer and an individual. I've quite enjoyed the process of doing the research and crafting it all together, and I hope I have managed to present the information in an interesting and easy to understand way.

If you could please take a brief moment to leave me an honest review of what you think of my book, I would greatly appreciate it. Your feedback is my only portal into the minds of my valued readers and is very important to me.

Head on over to my Amazon book page to leave a review. I would love to hear what you have to say.

Anyways, let's keep this journey moving. Happy reading!

A Note on Gut Health

One thing that was glaringly evident to me when I first started looking into the carnivore diet was the fact that there is, naturally, no fibre incorporated into the diet. Meat and other animal products contain no fibre, and seeing as how I thought fibre played such an important role in a healthy digestive system, I assumed there would definitely be some bathroom issues down the road. Yet, upon reading the stories and anecdotes from others on the diet, besides the occasional adjustment period right off the start, most seemed to be faring quite well with the reduction in dietary fibre intake. Not only that, but most were reporting that their digestion was actually improving over time when compared to their old diet. I decided to dig a bit further into why this may be, and I stumbled across some information that is actually rather interesting, as it goes against the conventional wisdom that fibre is the key to achieving regular, healthy bowel movements and a balanced digestive system.

It might help to give a quick definition and overview of fibre, just so we're all on the same page. Fibre is the carbohydrate portion of foods that we can't digest. Fibre only comes from plant foods, hence the lack of fibre in a 100% animal-based diet. Over the years it has generally been accepted that fibre aids digestive health by adding bulk (because we can't digest it) to our feces and help to prevent constipation and hemorrhoids.

That idea of fibre preventing constipation and promoting healthy bowel movements is probably one of the more popular tidbits of health related marketing that we are all exposed to. Just think of how many commercials, cereal boxes, bread bags, and granola bar packages you see advertising that they are high in fibre and "help to promote a healthy digestive system". At the very least, in Canada where I am from, it's quite common.

Turns out, there might not be much science supporting that claim. I actually managed to find a study that showed the complete opposite. In a study that was conducted on 63 individuals who were all experiencing constipation, the researchers tested the effectiveness of a low or no fibre diet on reducing the symptoms of the patient's constipation. The participants were instructed to first go on a no fibre diet for two weeks, then reduce their dietary fibre intake to a level they found comfortable. The researchers then measured their dietary fibre intake, constipation symptoms, and a few other markers at the one and six month marks.

At the six month mark, 41 of the individuals were still following the no fibre diet, 16 were on the reduced fibre diet, and the remaining 6 participants had resumed their high-fibre diet for personal or religious reasons. The results? The people who reduced or eliminated fibre from their diet experienced significant improvements in their digestive systems while the individuals who resumed their high-fibre diet had no change.

The individuals who stopped their dietary fibre intake completely had their average bowel movement frequency change from once every 3.75 days (with a standard deviation of 1.59 days) to once a day (with a standard deviation of 0 days).

The individuals who reduced their dietary intake, but did not eliminate it completely, had their average bowel movement frequency change from once every 4.19 days (with a standard deviation of 2.09 days) to once every 1.9 days (with a standard deviation of 1.21 days).

The individuals who remained on their high-fibre diet at the six month mark? Their average bowel movement frequency remained the same as it was at the time of the initial consultation. One movement, on average, every 6.83 days (with a standard deviation of 1.03 days).

The results also found that in the no fibre, reduced fibre, and high fibre groups the symptoms of bloating were 0%, 31.3% and 100%, and straining to pass stools occurred in 0%, 43.8%, and 100%, respectively.

In conclusion, the study summarized from these results that the symptoms of constipation can be effectively reduced by reducing or even eliminating fibre from your diet.

Now, this is only one study and as with a few other things in this book, I feel more research has to be done on this topic before we make any concrete assertions. But, with that being said, it does open the door to the idea that maybe what we have been told about the important role fibre plays in our digestive system isn't 100% accurate.

Couple this with the fact that there seems to be a wealth of anecdotal evidence online presenting people who are following a 100% animal-based diet who are not experiencing digestive health issues, and I think the case can be made that eating a diet void of fibre does not pose a risk to your digestive health. To the contrary, there might be a chance it could even improve it.

History of Animal-Based Diets

While it might seem like this idea of eating a diet mostly comprised of meat and animal products just recently popped into the world, as I just mentioned there are actually a few examples of groups of people eating this way (or close to it) for quite some time now.

Let's take a look at some of those groups of people, and dive in to what we know about how their diet might be impacting their overall health.

Inuit/Eskimo/Yupik

Referred to by a few different names depending on where you are from and who you are talking to, this group of people inhabits the northern expanses of Canada, the United States, Russia and Greenland. For simplicity's sake I will refer to them as Eskimo, only because it is the most commonly used term.

Eskimo typically inhabit Arctic or near-Arctic regions, and thus have adapted their way of life to deal with the long, cold, and harsh winters that are well known in those northernmost parts of the earth. They don't exactly have fresh fruits and vegetables popping up from the snow in the middle of the winter, so they have had to adopt a diet that revolves around the minimal types of foods that are available. Primarily, they eat a diet consisting of whale, seal, fish, moose, caribou and other varying types of seafood and land mammals. In essence, they subsist off of a very high-fat, high-protein, low-carbohydrate diet. Similar to that of the carnivore diet.

I say similar, and not the same, because while the vast majority of their diet is comprised of animal-based foods, the Eskimo will eat berries and other small plant matter in the summer months when available, making their diet not 100% animal-based. That being said, they are about as close to a carnivore diet as you can get.

Due to the fact that Eskimo eating habits are so irregular when compared to the typical Western diet, over the past hundred or so years multiple studies have been conducted in an effort to understand the health implications of their diet. More specifically, their cardiovascular health and their prevalence of heart disease.

Originally, many reports were coming out that talked about the incredibly low instances of heart disease amongst the Eskimo population. One researcher compared instances of "sclerosis" amongst a population of Eskimo from the Umanak region in North Greenland with that of an Eskimo population from Korpo, Finland. The Eskimos from Greenland followed a diet closer to the traditional Eskimo diet, while the group in Finland had begun to shift to a more Western diet. He found that at the time of the study—late 1940s—the rate of atherosclerotic disease was only 7.5% amongst the 1000 sampled individuals from the North Greenland Umanak Eskimos, which was about 2-3 times lower than that in Finland at the time.

This obviously made some waves in the health community, as it completely contradicted the conventional wisdom that a high-fat diet resulted in higher instances of heart disease. More follow up studies would inevitably have to be done in the following years to substantiate the claims that were being made.

A study was published in 2014 that aimed to shed some light on the debate concerning the link between the Eskimo diet and heart disease. The study looked back upon multiple studies that had been conducted over the previous 40 years in an attempt to draw some conclusions on the validity of the ideas being presented. The researchers concluded that based off the data in the studies, Greenland Eskimos and the Canadian and Alaskan Inuit actually have the same, if not higher, prevalence of coronary artery disease (CAD) as the non-Eskimo populations.

This makes it kind of confusing for someone from the outside looking in...One study is telling us that the Eskimo people have a 2-3 times lower instance of heart disease, while another is saying that it is actually the same if not higher. Who should we believe?

Well, one researcher has done us the favour of doing the analysis for us, in an effort to break down all of these studies and clear up some of the confusion. The researcher brings up a few solid ideas, one being that while recent studies may in fact point to the Eskimo and Inuit populations having the same, if not higher, prevalence of heart disease as the non-Eskimo population, they aren't following the same diet they originally were when the first studies were published. In particular, he points to the fact that the when the Eskimo diet was first measured in 1855 only 2-8% of their diet came from carbohydrates, whereas by 1970 it had climbed to 40%. Essentially, as the Eskimo groups became increasingly exposed to western culture they adopted the western diet in turn and gradually transitioned away from their traditional way of eating to more closely follow the typical western diet. This transition, although it can't be proven, is assumed to be responsible for the disparity in results from the studies as time went on. The Eskimos that were being studied in the 1970s were not following the same diet that the Eskimos were eating in the 1940s, or the Eskimos in the early 1900s. Most notably, the intake of refined sugar amongst the Greenland Eskimo in 1855 was only 6 grams/person/day, compared to 164-175 grams/person/day by the 1970s.

In short, the Eskimos who were originally studied followed a more traditional diet of primarily high-fat animal meats, while the Eskimos in the later studies were slowly shifting towards a diet that incorporated more refined sugars and carbohydrates. To put it in perspective, from 1855 to 1976 their intake of refined carbohydrates increased from 18/g per day (primarily obtained from bread) to 84-134/g per day (from bread, biscuits, and rye flour).

Now, it is important to point out that correlation doesn't necessarily mean causation, and we have to be careful when making assumptions. Simply put, just because two things are correlated—like the increase in consumption of carbohydrates, and the increase in the prevalence cardiovascular disease amongst Eskimo populations—does not mean that one caused the other.

But, if you want one man's opinion, I'd personally say it is safe to assume there is some relationship between the two. Which, if that holds to be true, could mean that the original studies are correct and a diet that is high in fat and low in carbohydrates can lead to lower instances of heart disease and improved cardiovascular health.

But, who knows...maybe it was a combination of many factors that all came together to give Eskimos those lower instances of heart disease. Maybe it was part genetics, part lifestyle, and part environment that all commingled together to create those health benefits, and not just diet alone.

If that is the case, it might help us to isolate the diet variable and look at another group of people that follow a similar diet—at least nutritionally speaking—yet live in a strikingly different environment, with some assumed variances in genetics, and a different lifestyle than the Eskimo.

Let's take a brief look at the East African hunter-gatherer tribes of the Maasai.

Maasai

Although historically the Maasai people lived across a much larger expanse of Africa, nowadays you can find the 900,000 or so tribespeople living mostly in southern Kenya and northern Tanzania. The Maasai are a semi-nomadic tribe that persists largely off livestock cultivation, and have gained popularity in recent years for some of the more unique elements of their nomadic lifestyle. In particular, there has been some buzz surrounding their almost exclusively animal-based diet.

The main staple in the diet of the Maasai is cow's milk. Closely followed by beef and cattle blood. They also throw in some fruits and vegetables when they are available—which is fairly rare—and if they're lucky enough to find it: honey. However, due to the fact that they are cattle ranchers, the vast majority of their diet comes from their cattle, and as I just mentioned, mainly in the form of milk. They will ferment the milk, make a type of yoghurt, mix it with bovine blood or just drink it plain. The consumption of beef is—surprisingly—fairly infrequent, as they typically reserve the eating of their cattle for special occasions. Their preferred meat is actually sheep or goat, but even that isn't normally consumed on a daily basis.

Considering that the Maasai don't actually consume a whole lot of meat, and their diet is largely comprised of milk, they might not seem like a great case study when looking at the carnivore diet. But, for the sake of discussing 100% animal-based diets, they do offer us some insight into a different approach on how that type of diet can be achieved. It doesn't just have to be steak all the time...

Despite the fact that the Maasai seem to eat a diet that is quite different from the aforementioned Eskimos of Greenland, they do share a similar type of nutritional intake as far as fats, carbs and proteins go. The Maasai, just like the Eskimo, subsist on a diet that predominantly contains high levels of fats and proteins, with proportionally lower levels of carbohydrates. In fact, the Maasai consume roughly two-thirds of their daily calories in the form of fats.

As far as health markers go, the Maasai—just like the Eskimo of the early 20th century—seem to have significantly low instance of cardiovascular disease, diabetes and obesity amongst their population when compared with Western populations. One study that looked at 400 Maasai men, women and children, found little to no clinical evidence of atherosclerosis (a disease where plaque builds up in your arteries) within the sample group. It also found that, despite a diet of mainly milk and meat, the men had no evidence for heart disease and actually had low levels of serum cholesterol.

The researchers in that study suggested a few potential explanations for their findings. One thought was that some type of protective mechanism was at play with the Maasai people. Meaning that something like their freedom from emotional stress or high levels of activity was protecting them from the adverse impacts a high fat diet would typically have on a population. This was just one possible reason they debated, however, in the end they did favour the conclusion that dietary fat is simply not responsible for coronary heart disease.

Now, just like the Eskimo, we can't be certain that it is their diet that keeps the Maasai population as healthy as they are. A staunch proponent of the carnivore diet might have you believe that they strictly have their diet to thank for their low prevalence of heart ailments and other lifestyle diseases. A naysayer might try to discount that and say it has everything to do with their genetics, lifestyle, and the population's ability to adapt over a long period of time to that particular diet. Personally, I think it is more than likely a combination of all those things.

First off, it is definitely important to point out that the Maasai are more active than the average American. It is a well-known fact that the more active you are, the better chance you have of having a properly functioning, healthy cardiovascular system. Turns out even just going for a leisurely walk can drastically improve your cardiovascular health, and reduce your risk of heart disease. And the Maasai walk. A lot.

Early on, some of the reports in the 1960s and 1970s that were coming out about the Maasai people mentioned that they were "very active", which could explain their low levels of heart disease and improved cardiovascular health. For most people reading those reports, the description of "very active" could have meant a few different things. Most people took it to mean that the Maasai were engaging in near athlete levels of physical activity on a regular basis: running for long distances on a consistent basis. That wasn't—and still isn't—the case.

Like I mentioned before, the Maasai actually spend a lot of their time walking. How do we know this? Well, a group of 370 Maasai were actually fitted with an extremely lightweight fitness tracker to measure their activity levels, then sent home and told to go about their normal lives for five days. The results showed that on average the Maasai move roughly 75% more than the average person in the West. Those increased activity levels are inevitably going to have some positive impact on their rates of heart disease and high cholesterol. But, how much of their health can be attributed to their activity levels and how much can be associated as a benefit of their diet?

This is just my personal opinion on the matter, but considering that there are many individuals (obviously not the majority) in our Western societies that match, if not exceed, the activity levels of the Maasai and still suffer from heart disease and high cholesterol, it might be safe to assume that there are some other factors at play here.

I'd like to think that based off the evidence from the studies, not only concerning the Maasai, but the Eskimo as well, that while it is definitely not the sole reason for their good health, there is a fairly strong case to be made that one of those factors could be diet.

Ten Day Get Started Meal Plan

Getting started is typically the hardest part with any new endeavour, especially a new diet. This is particularly true for the carnivore diet. That is why I decided to include a meal plan in this book. So that anyone who is looking to try out this new protocol can quickly jump right in, and not have to guess their way through the initial stages of the diet. Getting through the initial adjustment period can be quite hard for some people, and easier for others. Expect some fluctuation in your appetite, energy levels and potentially focus levels. Because of those potential impacts I found making sure I was getting enough sleep every night to be of utmost importance.

Now, this might not be a perfect meal plan but this is what I followed the first 10 days while I got started on the carnivore diet, and it seemed to work fairly well for me. As you'll notice, I tried to include a variety of different foods throughout the week and didn't just go straight to steak for every meal right off the hop. The goal of this meal plan was to help me gradually transition from a eating a variety of different foods, to eating only steak. However, if you would like to skip this meal plan all together and just hop straight in to eating only steak for every meal that is definitely an option.

Personally, I did find some value in this meal plan as it kept me more engaged with the diet off the start, and made the transition a bit easier.

A quick note: I didn't list water in the meal plan because I felt it would just get repetitive, but drink water. Lots of water.

This meal plan also includes some dairy, as I found it to help with the hunger right off the start while my body adjusted to the new way of eating. As I wasn't strictly eating fatty cuts of meat, the cheese was a good way to make sure I had enough fat in my meals. If you don't feel like including cheese in any of your meals, just simply remove it from the meal plan. I would however suggest keeping the butter in, as there really isn't too much of it and it is a great source of fat that really aids in the cooking process. Lastly, this meal plan is centered around my own lifestyle which is rather active and requires a fair amount of calories each day. If you find this is too much food for your lifestyle, simply scale back the suggested portions/serving sizes to better align with your needs.

Without further ado, the meal plan:

Day 1	
Breakfast	3 eggs (cooked with 1 tbsp grass fed butter) 4 slices bacon 2 slices cheese 1 cup coffee (Optional, preferably black)
Lunch	½ pound of ground beef ½ cup parmesan cheese (cooked with beef)
Supper	12 oz steak (Any cut will do, but try to go for a fattier cut like a ribeye) (cooked with 1 tbsp grass fed butter)

Day 2	

Breakfast	3 eggs (cooked with 1 tbsp grass fed butter) 4 slices bacon 2 slices cheese 1 cup coffee (Optional, preferably black)
Lunch	1 chicken breast 2 slices bacon ½ cup parmesan cheese (cooked on chicken) 1 cup bone broth
Supper	12 oz steak (cooked with 1 tbsp grass fed butter)

Day 3

Breakfast	3 eggs (cooked with 1 tbsp grass fed butter) 4 slices bacon 2 slices cheese 1 cup coffee (Optional, preferably black)
Lunch	12 oz steak (cooked with 1 tbsp grass fed butter)
Supper	Two fillets white fish (Basa, tilapia, etc.) 1 cup bone broth 2 slices cheese

Day 4	
Breakfast	3 eggs (cooked with 1 tbsp butter) 4 slices bacon 2 slices cheese 1 cup coffee (Optional, preferably black)
Lunch	½ pound ground turkey ½ cup parmesan cheese (cooked with turkey)
Supper	12 oz steak (cooked with 1 tbsp grass fed butter) 1 cup bone broth

Day 5	
Breakfast	3 eggs (cooked with 1 tbsp grass fed butter) 4 slices bacon 2 slices cheese 1 cup coffee (Optional, preferably black)
Lunch	12 oz steak (cooked with 1 tbsp grass fed butter)

Supper	½ pound ground beef ½ cup parmesan cheese (cooked with beef)

Day 6

Breakfast	3 eggs (cooked with 1 tbsp butter) 4 slices bacon 2 slices cheese 1 cup coffee (Optional, preferably black)
Lunch	10 oz steak (cooked with 1 tbsp grass fed butter)
Supper	12 oz steak (cooked with 1 tbsp grass fed butter)

Day 7

Breakfast	3 eggs (cooked with 1 tbsp butter) 4 slices bacon 2 slices cheese 1 cup coffee (Optional, preferably black)
Lunch	12 oz steak (cooked with 1 tbsp grass fed butter)

Supper	12 oz steak (cooked with 1 tbsp grass fed butter)

Day 8	
Breakfast	10 oz steak (cooked with 1 tbsp grass fed butter)
Lunch	10 oz steak (cooked with 1 tbsp grass fed butter)
Supper	10 oz steak (cooked with 1 tbsp grass fed butter)

Day 9	
Breakfast	10 oz steak (cooked with 1 tbsp grass fed butter)
Lunch	8 oz steak (cooked with 1 tbsp grass fed butter)
Supper	8 oz steak (cooked with 1 tbsp grass fed butter)

Day 10	
Breakfast	10 oz steak (cooked with 1 tbsp grass fed butter)
Lunch	8 oz steak (cooked with 1 tbsp grass fed butter)
Supper	8 oz steak (cooked with 1 tbsp grass fed butter)

Important Notes/Tips

- Make sure you are getting 7-9 hours sleep every night to help maintain energy levels
- If you find yourself about to cheat off the plan, don't go too far off the deep end (Ex: cookies, breads, fast food). Settle for something like real peanut butter that is high in protein and fat, and relatively low in sugars.
- Cheese is a great snack if you find yourself dying of hunger.
- The key is keeping your diet high in fat and protein while limiting carbohydrate intake as much as possible. The fat is important as it will help to keep you feeling full longer and provide much needed calories, this diet won't work if you only eat lean meats.
- Be prepared for changes in your appetite. Some days you might not feel hungry for 10 hours, others you may feel like eating everything in the house. Listen to your body and don't force feed or starve yourself.

How to Keep Costs Down

Eating an all-meat diet can be expensive. Just think of your typical grocery list. What is the most expensive item on it? Usually the meat.

Now, I think most would agree that you can't put a price on your health. If you're going to spend a few extra dollars on one aspect of your life, health and well-being seems like a worthy choice to me. That being said, you might not revel in the idea of your monthly grocery bill doubling as you stock up on expensive ribeye steaks. While it is impossible to get around the fact that meat is just plain expensive, there are a few little tips and tricks you can employ to ensure you are getting the biggest bang-for-your-buck.

Tip #1) Buy marked down products

This first tip might seem like a bit of a no-brainer, but it is easily the best way to save money on this diet. Many grocery stores will mark down their meats anywhere from 25-75% off a day or two before they are set to expire. This can translate into huge savings for you.

You might have some trepidations in buying meat that will expire soon, and rightfully so. No one wants to get sick. The best way to get around this is to either cook the meat the same day you buy it, or put it straight into the freezer when you get home. I typically buy myself 2-3 days worth of food when I shop, cook one day worth of meals right when I get home and then freeze the rest.

It is also important to note that you won't find marked down products at all times when you visit the grocery store. Many stores will have a certain day where they go out and mark items down for a quick sale (I found my usual grocery store does this every Tuesday morning), while others might do it every morning at a certain time. Simply go up to the butcher/meat department at your grocery store and ask them when they tend to go mark down the meat. Then simply make sure to get to the grocery store early on those days to take advantage of the slashed down prices.

Tip #2) Specialty grocery stores

This one can be hit-or-miss. However, it can be worth it to check out some specialty grocery stores and markets to potentially find certains types of meat priced differently.

People have reported that certain specialty grocery stores can sell some types of meat for much cheaper than you'll find at typical grocery stores. While I haven't explored this extensively myself, I have heard rumblings of it on a few different blogs. One example given was finding pork belly at a Korean market for up to $7.99/lb while at an Italian grocery store being able to buy pork belly for $2.99/lb.

I myself do not eat much pork belly—my pork consumption begins and ends with bacon—but even so, I imagine this principle may hold true for some other types of meat. It could be worth exploring.

Tip #3) Cut out the middleman

This one may be my favourite. It has one important requirement though, a big freezer.

If you have a large freezer you can use, one of the best ways to save money on beef is to go straight to the source and find a rancher/farmer to buy a cow. When you eliminate the cost of having to buy the beef from a company who has to factor in the cost of shipping the cow, butchering it, shipping it back to grocery stores, then marking it up for a profit, there are great savings to be had. You also have the added benefit of knowing exactly where your meat came from, how it was raised, and what it was fed.

If you go on any type of online sale website: Craigslist, Kijiji, etc. you can look for local farmers selling cows. If you purchase the cow straight from them, your cost per pound of beef is drastically reduced. After that you simply pay to get it butchered and freeze all the meat. Even after buying the cow and paying to get it butchered you will still be saving a big chunk of change. You might even get lucky and find an experienced rancher/farmer willing to do the butchering for you themselves for a smaller fee than an actual butcher would charge.

If the larger upfront cost is an issue, you could always consider splitting the cost of the cow with a family member or friend. You could really split it with as many people as you like. This would help to get the upfront cost smaller.

Tip #4) Start hunting

I'll admit this might not be the easiest or most reasonable way for most people to save money on their meat. It is however, a nice benefit of hunting. You could end up getting yourself a few hundred pounds of elk to stock into the freezer. This concept is really a continuation of buying the cow from the rancher...cut out the middleman and go straight to the source. This also comes with the added benefit of you knowing that your meat is from a wild, naturally fed animal free of any added hormones.

Now, there are obviously many costs associated with hunting (equipment, tags, licenses, etc.). But, maybe a family member/friend already hunts and you can try to tag along with them and share some equipment.

Wrapping It Up

When I first heard rumblings of this new all-meat carnivore diet I—like most—was skeptical to say the least. It challenged much of what I thought I understood of nutrition and what it meant to eat a healthy diet. Nonetheless, I decided to give it a fair chance and did my best to examine it objectively. Through the process of engaging with this diet myself and doing the research to put this book together, I came to a few personal conclusions on this way of eating. In the end these are just my opinions and I could very well be wrong, but if you want my two cents, here's what I think.

First off, I think a lot of the benefits people are experiencing have less to do with what they **are** eating and more to do with what they **aren't** eating. It's the subtraction of foods and not the addition of only meat that is contributing to most of the positive health improvements. If you were to take the average person eating the typical Western diet and transition them to a 100% animal-based diet, doesn't it only make sense they would see some drastic benefits? Think of what they're cutting out. No more chips and soda, or muffins and fast food. Just moving away from a diet that is riddled with sugar, processed foods and empty calories is bound to have a positive impact on your health and weight.

On top of that, when you eat 100% animal-based you are taking in significantly less calories than you normally are on a traditional diet. You aren't losing weight because meat has some magic weight loss properties, you're losing weight because you're eating a lot less calories than you usually do. As much as people might complicate the subject of weight loss, in the end it really comes down to a simple formula:

Calories burned > calories consumed = weight loss.

Or in other words, if you burn more calories than you take in you will lose weight.

Now, obviously everyone is different but let's say that the average person eats around 2500-3000 calories a day on their typical diet. An individual who eats a relatively healthy diet might be closer to the 2500 mark, while someone who eats a lot of junk food (chips, soda, candy bars, fast food) is most likely well above the 3000 level. In fact, according to The Food and Agriculture Organization, Americans eat an average of 3,600 calories per day. If they move to a diet where they are eating 2-3 ribeye steaks per day and only drinking water, their daily caloric intake is going to drop significantly. A normal 8 ounce ribeye steak is going to sit at around 650-700 calories on average. If you eat 3 in a day, you'd be lucky to crack the 2000 calorie threshold. This drop in calories is most likely the main contributor to the drastic weight loss people are reporting on this diet. It also might just be responsible for a lot of the other health benefits being experienced.

A number of studies have looked at the impact calorie restriction can have on a person's health. One randomized controlled trial conducted in March of 2018 found that in a sample population of 53 healthy, non-obese men and women aged 21-50, those who reduced their caloric intake by 15% over the course of 2 years experienced decreased systemic oxidative stress and lost an average of 9 kilograms of body weight. All of this happened despite not following a specific diet or having weight loss as the goal of the study. They also found that cutting caloric intake slowed signs of aging and metabolism, protected against age-related diseases, and led to general improvements in mood and health-related quality of life. This conclusion was closely mimicked by another study which looked at the relationship between caloric restriction and inflammatory diseases. The study found that reducing caloric intake appears to consistently protect against chronic inflammatory diseases such as cardiovascular disease and diabetes.

So, what does that all mean in the context of the carnivore diet? Well, just one of the aforementioned points on its own doesn't account for all the amazing benefits people are experiencing on this diet. However, combine them together and I personally think we paint a pretty good picture of what is going on here.

People are cutting out the unhealthy elements of their diet such as sugar, processed foods and refined carbohydrates while simultaneously restricting their calories to end up with a caloric deficit. Both of these things are coming together to drastically reduce inflammation in the body, help the individual lose weight, and improve their general feeling of health and wellbeing.

In the end, I'll leave it for you to decide if the carnivore diet is right for you. Hopefully over the course of this book I've given enough information to help you navigate through the ever complicated landscape of nutrition and diet, and to help you make your own decision on if this diet is right for you.

Now, for anyone thinking of switching over to the carnivore diet I would like to offer one little piece of advice: get your bloodwork done. As I have mentioned a time or two throughout this book, everyone is different in the way they respond to things. This diet could be perfect for one person, and a disaster for the next. That is why it is important to tread carefully and ensure you are tracking your health as you make any changes. Get your bloodwork done before you start on this diet, then again a few months in to see how your body is doing with the changes. It might seem like a big hassle or a bit of overkill, but it can provide you with some concrete evidence to see how your body is changing alongside your diet.

Again, if you'd like to read further into any of the resources or studies within this book I have provided links within the Additional Resources chapter.

Making the Meals

Let's face it...a recipe guide for a diet that only allows the consumption of meat and animal products is going to be pretty one dimensional, just by nature of the limits within the diet. If you plan on sticking to this diet 100% and being strict to not include dairy, then the types of recipes you can follow are severely limited. For those people, in lieu of elaborate recipes I will provide you with some of—what I have found to be—the best ways to prepare your standard carnivore meals. How to cook your steaks for optimal tenderness and flavour. How prepare your own bone broth. The best way to cook marrow/soup bones. Along with a few other preparation techniques for other staple meals.

Now, if you plan on including some dairy in your diet and maybe allowing for the odd sauce to enter into the mix, your ability to experiment with recipes expands slightly. For those people, I will include some simple and easy to make recipes that I have found to work great. They might not belong on the menu of any 5-star restaurants or pass the scrupulous taste gauntlet of Gordon Ramsay, but if you're looking to add a bit of variety into your diet and get away from simple steaks, they offer some solace.

Basic Recipes/Cooking Methods

The Best Way to Cook a Steak (The Reverse Sear Method)

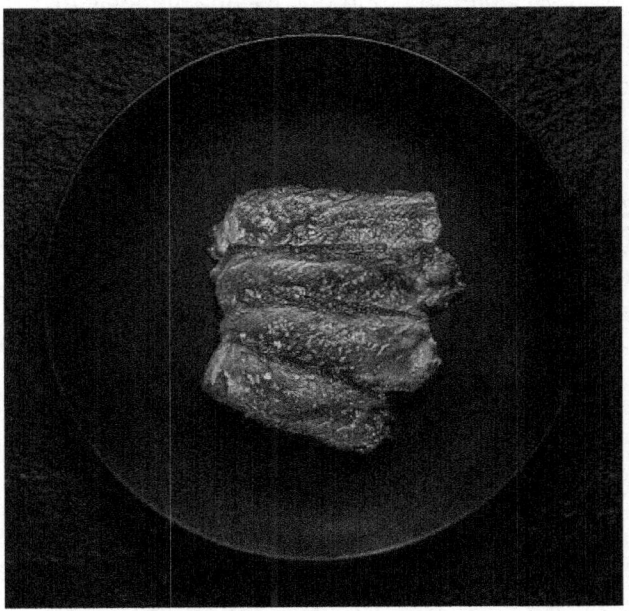

You're going to be eating a lot of steak on this diet so you better know how to cook one. You can throw it on the barbeque, fry it in a pan, cook it in the oven or do it any way you please if you have a different favourite method. In my opinion, however, the best way to cook a steak is with the reverse-sear method. Here is how to do it:

1) Preheat your oven to 425 degrees Fahrenheit.
2) Get yourself a ribeye steak at least 1" thick (can be done with any cut of steak).

3) Salt and pepper your steak to taste.
4) Put your steak on a tin foil lined pan (easier to clean up).
5) Put your steak in the oven.
    a) Depending on how well cooked you like your steak, the time you leave it in the oven will vary.
    b) I personally prefer a medium rare steak (as will most people), and find that leaving the steak to cook for around 10-12 minutes in the oven works best. If you want it cooked more, leave it in longer, if you prefer a rarer steak, take it out earlier.
6) While the steak is in the oven, put 2 tbsp of grass fed butter into a pan and get it going on high heat.
7) Take your steak out when it has reached your desired doneness, and transfer to the pan.
8) Sear the steak for 1 minute on each side, only flipping it once.
9) Remove the steak from the pan and place on a plate, cover it in foil and let it rest for 10 minutes.
10) After the steak has rested for 10 minutes, enjoy!

Easy Oven Roast

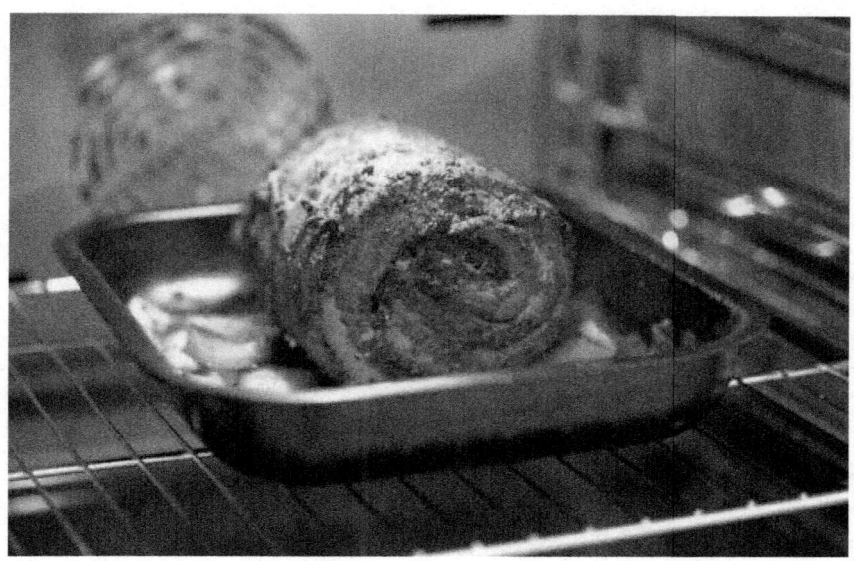

Although roast isn't all that common on this diet, I did try it a few times simply because I stumbled across a great deal at the grocery store. Here is how to do a simple oven roast:

1) Preheat your oven to 375 degrees Fahrenheit
2) If your roast is untied, tie it at 3" intervals with some cotton twine
3) Place your roast in an oven safe pan
4) Season your roast with ½ teaspoon of salt, ½ teaspoon of ground black pepper, and ½ teaspoon garlic powder.
5) Roast in oven for 20 minutes per pound of meat
6) Remove and cover with foil, let rest for 15-20 minutes and enjoy!

Marrow Bones

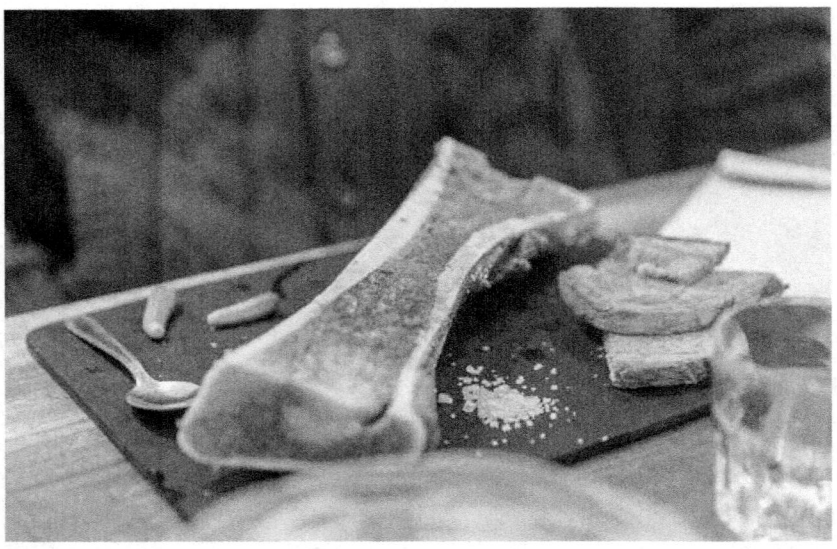

This was one thing I had never tried before this diet, and I had some trepidations with eating bone marrow. Turns out that hesitation was unwarranted. This easy recipe has turned out to be one of my favourites:

1) Preheat your oven to 450 degrees Fahrenheit
2) Place the bones on a tin foil lined baking sheet
3) Bake in the oven for 15 minutes
4) Turn the oven to broil and keep an eye on the bones until they are golden brown on the top
5) Remove from the oven and salt and pepper
6) Use a spoon to scoop out the marrow and enjoy!

Making Your Own Bone Broth

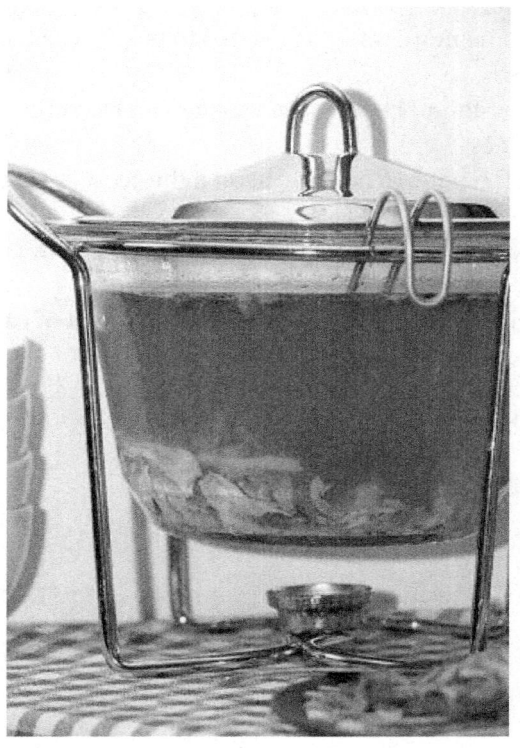

While the general idea of making a bone broth is pretty straightforward: boil some bones in water. I figured I would still breakdown the easiest method for you guys. Here it is:

1) Get a large pot and fill it with 3.75 litres of water
2) Add in a half cup of apple cider vinegar (this helps draw out the minerals from the bones)

3) Place roughly 3-4 pounds of beef marrow and knuckle bones in the pot, as well as 2 pounds of meaty bones (such as short ribs).
4) Add some more water as needed to ensure the bones are all covered.
5) Let it sit for an hour so the vinegar can leech the minerals from the bones
6) Bring the pot to a boil and scrape the scum from the top of the water
7) Reduce to a simmer and leave it for 24-72 hours (the longer the better).
8) After it is done, ensure all the marrow is out of each bone and drain the broth into a separate container.
9) Store it in a fridge for 5 to 7 days or in the freezer for up to 6 months.

Bacon Wrapped Scallops

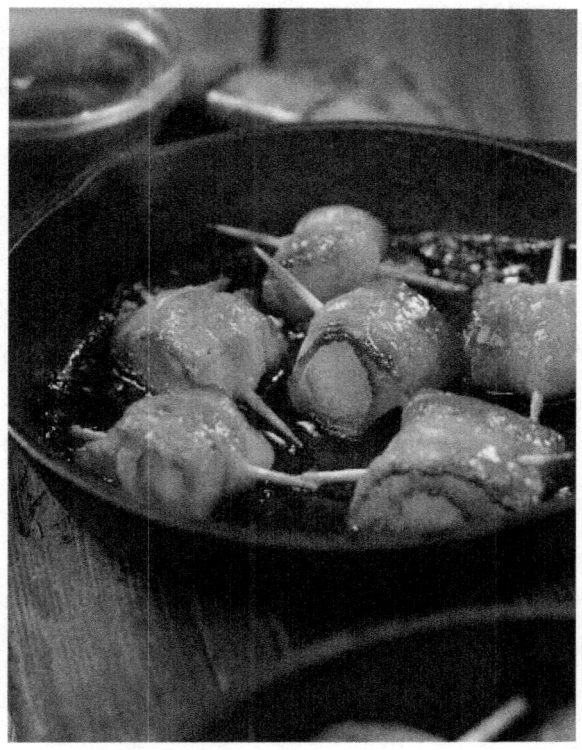

I like to throw some variety into my diet every now and then. These are a perfect—and easy—way to add something delicious and different into your carnivore diet when you're feeling bored.

1) Preheat oven to 425 degrees Fahrenheit.
2) Defrost scallops if frozen, and pat them dry with some paper towel.
3) Wrap each scallop with a half slice (or full if you really want) of bacon and secure with a toothpick.
4) Drizzle some olive oil lightly over the tops of the scallops.

5) Salt and pepper to taste.
6) Spread the scallops out on a baking sheet lined with tin foil or parchment paper.
7) Bake in the oven for 12-15 minutes depending on how big your scallops are.

More Inclusive Recipes

Eggs With Cheese and Bacon

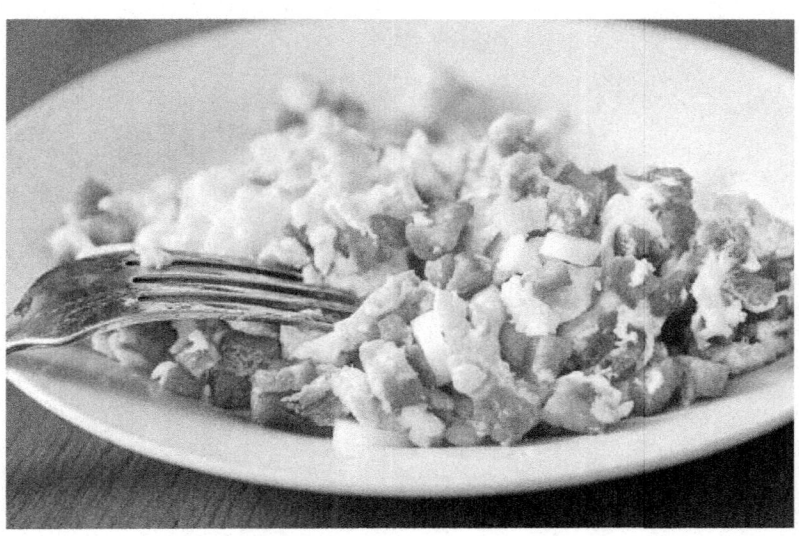

Alright, this once is a really simple recipe but has been one of my go-to breakfasts for a long time. There is a reason bacon and eggs have stuck around as a breakfast staple for so long.

1) Heat 2 tablespoons of coconut oil in a pan on medium heat
2) Crack 3 eggs into the pan once coconut oil is heated
3) Stir the eggs and coconut oil until eggs are well mixed
4) Continually stir with a spatula until eggs are scrambled and fluffy
5) Cut up 3 slices of bacon into small pieces and mix with eggs
6) Salt and pepper to taste
7) Grate ⅓ cup of cheese (cheddar or parmesan are best) on eggs
8) Stir and mix the cheese with the eggs

9) Continue to cook for 3-5 minutes then remove from pan

Slow Cooker Roast

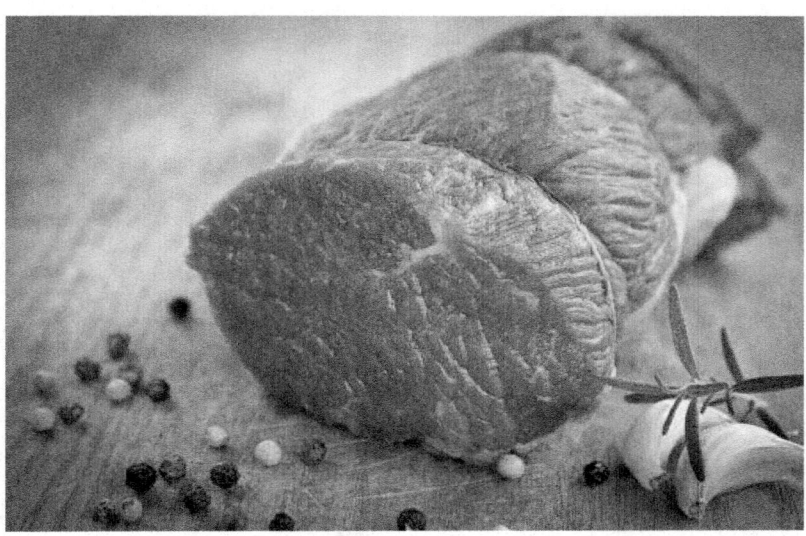

Slow cooking is a great way to take some tougher cuts of meat and cook them down to a softer and juicier tenderness. Plus it is simple and convenient. Throw a roast in the slow cooker before you leave for the day and when you get home you'll have supper waiting for you.

1) Take 4 pound chuck roast and rub a generous amount of salt and pepper around the outside
2) Heat up 2 tablespoons of canola oil in a large skillet or pan
3) Brown all sides in the pan on high heat, for roughly 4 minutes per side.
4) Take roast and transfer to slow cooker pot
5) Add 2 cups beef broth, 2 tablespoons soy sauce, and 1 tbsp red chilli flakes to the slow cooker pot
6) Cook on low for 8 hours
7) With one hour left, mix 2 tablespoons of cornstarch with 2 tablespoons of water. Pour into the pot and mix with the broth.
8) Cover and let cook for remaining hour.

Ground Beef

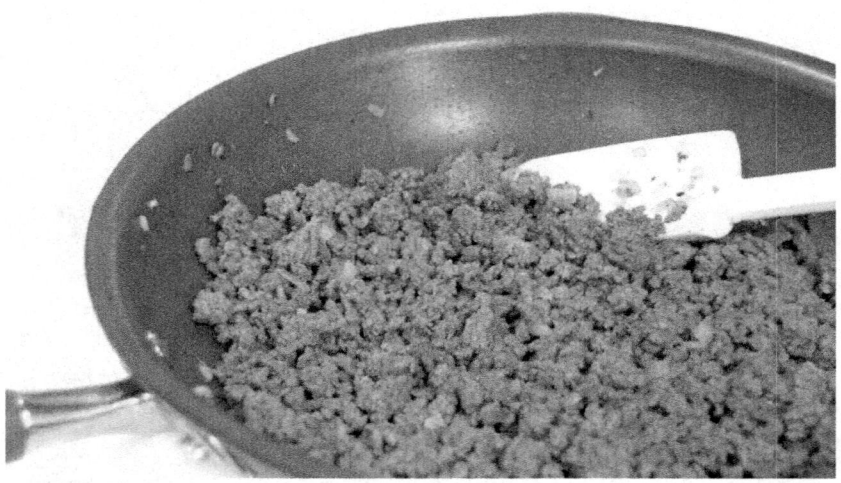

Plain ground beef is fine and all, but just adding a few simple ingredients can improve the overall dish drastically.

1) Defrost ground beef if frozen.
2) Heat 2 tablespoons of canola oil in a medium pan or skillet.
3) Mince 2 cloves garlic and throw in the pan with the oil.
4) Fry the garlic in the oil until fragrant.
5) Add 1.5-2 lbs of ground beef to the pan.
6) Break up the beef into smaller pieces as it cooks for 3 minutes.
7) Cover the pan with a lid and cook for 5-7 minutes, stirring occasionally.
8) Remove the lid and cook for another 5 minutes.
9) Add ½ cup parmesan cheese
10) Stir and cook for 1 minute
11) Remove from pan and enjoy!

Grilled White Fish

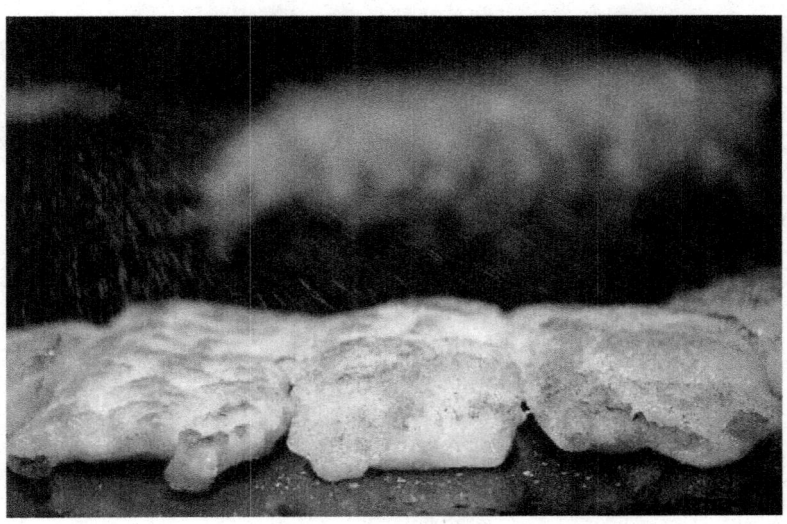

It might not be the best meal all on its own due to the low fat content in white fish, but it is a quick and easy way to throw in some variety if you're craving something other than beef. One of the best parts of this recipe is that you can simply cook the fish straight from frozen with no issues, no need to wait for anything to defrost.

1) Heat up 2 tbsp butter in a pan on medium heat
2) Salt and pepper your frozen fish (I prefer basa, but tilapia, cod, or sole works too)
3) Place in pan and cook for around 5 minutes on the first side, or until lightly browned
4) Flip and cook the other side, add 1 tbsp more butter if necessary to prevent sticking
5) Add in some red chilli flakes if you'd like at this point
6) Continue to cook until both sides are lightly browned
7) Remove from pan and enjoy!

Stir Fry Steak

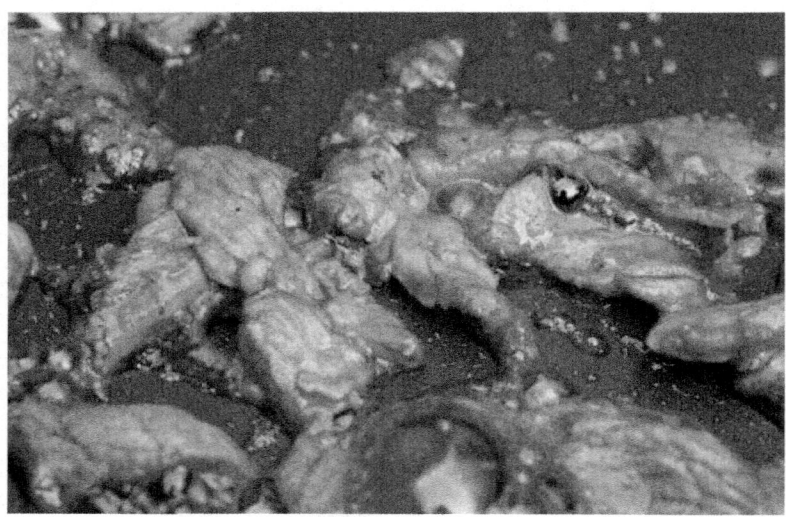

Grilling up a ribeye steak is definitely my favourite way to eat beef. But every now and then I like to do things differently. My other favourite method is simply stir frying some smaller strips of steak. With a few simple ingredients, this stir fry is a great change up from your usual steak.

1) Heat up 2 tablespoons canola oil in a pan over medium heat
2) Mince 2 cloves garlic and add to pan
3) Fry the garlic until fragrant
4) Add in sliced beef to pan
5) Grind some fresh ground pepper over the beef
6) Add in 1 tbsp Worchester sauce
7) Cook the beef for roughly 5 minutes
8) Make sure not to cook the beef until it is completely grey...think of trying to cook a medium rare steak.
9) Remove from pan and enjoy!

Additional Resources

The Evolution of the Human Diet
http://www.immpressmagazine.com/the-evolution-of-diet/

The Western Diet and Lifestyle and Disease
https://www.dovepress.com/the-western-diet-and-lifestyle-and-diseases-of-civilization-peer-reviewed-article-RRCC

Origins and evolution of the Western diet: health implications for the 21st century
https://academic.oup.com/ajcn/article/81/2/341/4607411

Sugar consumption now vs 100 years ago
http://www.divineeatingout.com/food-1/sugar-consumption-now-vs-100-years-ago

What the world eats?
https://www.nationalgeographic.com/what-the-world-eats/

Stopping or reducing dietary fibre intake reduces constipation and its associated symptoms
https://www.ncbi.nlm.nih.gov/pmc/articles/PMC3435786/

Low-carbohydrate diet on low-grade inflammation in type 2 diabetes
https://www.ncbi.nlm.nih.gov/pmc/articles/PMC4025600/

Calorie restricted, high-fat diet on obese subjects
https://www.ncbi.nlm.nih.gov/pmc/articles/PMC3845365/

Effects of dietary fat on testosterone in men
https://www.ncbi.nlm.nih.gov/pubmed/8942407

Weight loss with a low-carbohydrate, Mediterranean, or low-fat diet
https://www.nejm.org/doi/full/10.1056/NEJMoa0708681

Low carbohydrate vs conventional weight loss diet in obese adults
http://annals.org/aim/fullarticle/717452

How eating meat made us human
http://time.com/4252373/meat-eating-veganism-evolution/

Average person consumes 300% more sugar than recommended
http://naturalsociety.com/sugar-the-toxicity-question-and-what-to-do-about-it/

Added sugar intake and cardiovascular diseases mortality among US adults
https://jamanetwork.com/journals/jamainternalmedicine/fullarticle/1819573

Dietary sugars and body weight: systematic review and meta-analyses
https://www.ncbi.nlm.nih.gov/pubmed/23321486

Sugar-sweetened beverages and risk of obesity and type 2 diabetes
https://www.ncbi.nlm.nih.gov/pubmed/20138901

International study of macro/micronutrients and blood pressure
https://www.ncbi.nlm.nih.gov/pubmed/21357284

Dietary protein intake and kidney function
https://www.ncbi.nlm.nih.gov/pmc/articles/PMC1262767/

A new dietary allowance for Vitamin C based on antioxidant and health effects in humans
https://academic.oup.com/ajcn/article/69/6/1086/4714888

90 days on the carnivore diet: results and insights
https://medium.com/@andylindquist/90-days-on-a-carnivore-diet-results-and-insights-8d07692869fe

Setting dietary intake levels: problems and pitfalls
https://www.ncbi.nlm.nih.gov/pubmed/17913222

Ascorbic acid and the immune system
http://www.orthomolecular.org/library/jom/2005/pdf/2005-v20n03-p179.pdf

Prolonged meat diets with a study of kidney function and ketosis (1930)
http://www.jbc.org/content/87/3/651.full.pdf

Which dietary reference intake is best suited to serve as a basis for nutrition labeling?
https://academic.oup.com/jn/article/136/10/2457/4746679

Medical studies in North Greenland 1948-1949
https://www.ncbi.nlm.nih.gov/pubmed/14884934?dopt=Abstract

Eskimos and heart disease: facts or wishful thinking?
https://www.ncbi.nlm.nih.gov/pubmed/25064579?dopt=Abstract

Increase in the intake of refined carbohydrates and sugars may have led to health decline in Greenland Eskimos
https://openheart.bmj.com/content/3/2/e000444.full#ref-1

The composition of food consumed by Greenland Eskimos
https://www.ncbi.nlm.nih.gov/pubmed/961471?dopt=Abstract

Cardiovascular disease in the Maasai
https://www.atherosclerosis-journal.com/article/S0368-1319(64)80041-7/abstract

The Maasai keep healthy despite a high fat diet
http://sciencenordic.com/maasai-keep-healthy-despite-high-fat-diet

Stopping or reducing dietary fibre intake reduces constipation and its associated symptoms
https://www.ncbi.nlm.nih.gov/pmc/articles/PMC3435786/

Calorie restriction trial in humans suggests benefits for age-related diseases
https://www.sciencedaily.com/releases/2018/03/180322141008.htm

Calorie restriction and chronic inflammatory diseases
https://www.ncbi.nlm.nih.gov/pmc/articles/PMC3193874/

All Rights Reserved

© 2018 Kent Dixon

Printed in Dunstable, United Kingdom